THE QIGONG REJUVENATION DIET WITH BREATHING AND 14 MOVEMENTS

An Integrated Method for Health and Wellness

Keiko Murakumo
Translated by Joel Challender

authorHOUSE®

AuthorHouse™ UK Ltd.
500 Avebury Boulevard
Central Milton Keynes, MK9 2BE
www.authorhouse.co.uk
Phone: 08001974150

First published by AuthorHouse   7/21/2008

ISBN: 978-1-4343-7901-6 (e)
ISBN: 978-1-4343-7900-9 (sc)

Printed in the United States of America
Bloomington, Indiana

This book is printed on acid-free paper.

PREFACE

Around the world, a great many books have been written about Qi Gong, but it is often said that the more you try and understand what is written in them, the more confused you get. This is because Qi Gong is something that cannot be experienced only from reading books and acquiring knowledge. It is only when we practice Qi Gong that we start to unravel its true essence.

Presently, a great many people on this planet suffer from hunger yet at the same time a great many others are stricken by a problem of excess or inappropriate consumption, a condition that manifests as obesity. Indeed, this issue of excess energy is not only limited to humans, but extends to a swelling population and to so many environmental problems. It is a problem that can be seen as occurring on a planetary level. If we look at ourselves in the same way as our planet, in terms of a life-form, we can surely see that we have become unbalanced.

It could also be said that while we have brought this natural cataclysm upon ourselves, we are also in the midst of a natural healing process, trying to redress the balance that we have upset. It is my belief that if we as individuals commit ourselves to improving things on the level of our own personal physical environment, these efforts would eventually translate into improving the earth on a macro level.

I wrote this book with the aim of enabling the reader to quickly incorporate a practical self healing health care into their lives. I firmly hope that this book will act as a tool for you to use for improving your health, and lead to your self-development.

TABLE OF CONTENTS

INTRODUCTION

In this book, prior to discovering Qigong Dieting and the 14 practical methods of Qigong, I would first like to explain the perception of Qi (vital energy) and aura from the point of view of classic traditional medicine. Though the written word cannot well express the composition and effect of invisible Qi, through putting some time into studying how people from ancient times perceived the energy centers that are the cosmos and the human body we can gain a better appreciation of the meaning of practicing Qigong, and discover a sense of the new from the ancient. Reaching this essential understanding, we will be able to discover a novel way of looking at one's own body and health.

CHINESE MEDICINE

People in ancient times perceived that the life energy known as Qi governs all phenomenon and substance in the universe, believing that everything is born due to changes in Qi. This notion was applied to the human body in China's oldest medical books, written between 202 BC and 8 AD, which had it that within Qi there are positive and a negative energies ("yin and yang") and if these are balanced one is in a healthy condition; when unbalanced, one is an unhealthy state. These dual concepts of yin and yang originate in ancient Chinese philosophy, which describe two primal opposing but complementary principles or cosmic forces said to be found in all non-static objects and processes in the universe. Examples of the relationship between ying and yang are, the moon and the sun, water and fire, night and day. Yin and Yang possess anathematic qualities, but rather than repelling against each other, they act as a balance to ensure that the force of one side does not become too strong. For example, fire cancels out water, and in turn water is evaporated by fire. The relationship of Ying and Yang is also one of aiding one another,

Channels in the body through which Qi flows are known as meridians. In "The New Medicine of the Mind: Healing without Freud or Prozac", (2005) Dr.David Servan-Schreiber describes meridians as *"'virtual' lines running up and down the body that had been described 2,500 years ago. Meridians do not correspond to any material reality in the body, such as the arterial and venous systems, or the lymphatic ducts, or even the dermatomes. Yet they were so clearly manifest in my own body"*

These meridians are the 14 principal pathways that run energy, blood, saliva, hormones and urine through the body, reciprocally interlinking each and every part. There are points situated along these passages, which are linked to various bodily functions including muscles and internal organs, and while there are points aside from those in these passages, it is said there are 720 major places where points are located. People whose pathways and points are in a good condition are healthy, and people with blocked or hindered pathways are unhealthy. Incidentally, if pressed from outside the skin, these points induce a piercing-type pain and a languid, drowsy sensation.

Apart from Ying and Yang, another principal notion underpinning Chinese medicine is the doctrine of the five elements. In traditional Chinese philosophy, natural phenomena can be classified into the Five Elements of wood, fire, earth, metal and water, and these elements were used for describing interactions and relationships between all phenomena, physical and non-physical.

Gogyo(five element)

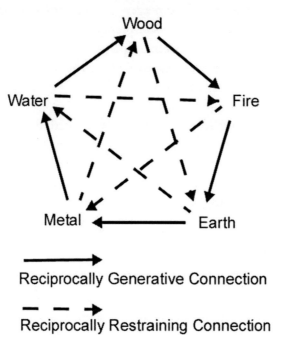

Reciprocally Generative Connection

Reciprocally Restraining Connection

Acupuncture, moxibustion (a traditional Chinese medicine technique that involves the burning of mugwort, a small, spongy herb, to facilitate healing), herbal medicine, pressure point massage (Shiatsu) and other kinds of massage are among some of the treatments recommended by others to restore stagnant life energy and improve health.

PRESSURE POINTS INDICATE ILLNESS

Before the dawn of modern medical diagnosing technology, Chinese doctors would diagnose a patient's condition by the color and form of their skin, eyes and tongue, and by taking their pulse with the fingertips. Doctors can gauge a lot of information from pressure points because with illness, toxins, stress and discomfort accumulate in the pressure points, and materialize as inflammation, blockage and swelling. In fact these diagnostic methods are still employed today, and illness can be predicted in advance rather than being detected by machine.

Consider as an example an incident that took place before me at a hospital in Peking that combined Eastern and Western Medicine. One day, a patient was carried into the emergency ward complaining of stomach pain, and just as the surgeons were preparing to investigate his condition with an ultrasound examination a professor of acupuncture who happened to be in the vicinity examined the patient's ear and diagnosed acute appendicitis, after which they went immediately into surgery.

While I was studying acupuncture and moxibustion at this hospital, a woman sitting next to me on the bench in the waiting room suddenly lost consciousness and passed out. I was astonished to witness a Chinese Doctor reviving her by simply sticking one needle onto the pressure point that heals fainting.

INDIAN AYURVEDIC MEDICINE AND QIGONG CONNECTION

Ayurveda from the sophisticated ancient Indian civilization has a lot in common with Chinese medicine. It is believed that during the classical period of Ayuverda, from 1700BC to 700AD, Ayurveda and Marma therapy spread across Eastern China and into Japan.

Ayurveda, which literally means "the science of life", is an ancient system of health care native to the Indian Subcontinent, and is rich in subtle knowledge and wisdom that enables healthy living through therapeutic measures like Yoga that relate to physical, mental, social and spiritual harmony.

In India, life energy is referred to as "prahna", and the treatment similar to acupuncture is known as Marma. In Marma therapy there are 107 main pressure points, and then apart from this some minor points. Marma is the vital tool in Yoga and Ayurvedic medicine. The rivers stretched around the body through which prahna flows are called "nadi", and as with the meridians, there are a total of 14 altogether.

When the body is off-kilter, the supply of prahna is hindered and lacking, so using pressure, heat, minerals, herbs and aroma oils it is possible to restore the flow of prahna and marma to the original state. This treatment can help deal with nearly any ailment and injury, including rheumatism, gout, chronic internal diseases, neuralgia, stoke-induced paralysis, and psychosis.

Hatha Yoga, a training in conjunction with Ayurveda, has been practiced from as far back as 3000BC, and one of the aims of the poses (asana) one adopts in Hatha Yoga is to loosen and broaden the range of motion of the articular ligaments as much as possible, making a supple body, and enabling prahna (life-sustaining force, vital energy) to flow properly into the various Marma areas of the body.

In the background to Ayurveda are the original 3 gunas (abstractly meaning "qualities") of Samkhya philosophy, are a way of describing the powers or tendencies of energy• tamas (inertia, darkness, lethargy), rajasu (dynamism, action, motion) and satva (lucidity, balance, purity). Then there are the 5 main elements which are from the central concepts of Yoga and Ayurveda, namely earth, water, fire, wind, and sky.

Reverting to the subject of the human body, within our bodies are 7 main energy pivots called Chakras. Chakra means "circle of light" in Sanskrit, and refers to energy centers located along the backbone. Through coil-like revolution, each of these chakras generates their own electromagnetic field, and through catenation with other chakras create aura. Auras in turn have a characteristic in terms of their color, shape, size, magnitude and the way they revolve and circulate. Chakras each bind with a respective endocrine gland and principal plexus, and on absorbing life energy / prahna, segments it into different components and along the nadi, transmit raw live energy to the body by sending it into the nervous and endocrine and systems and the blood.

In ancient times and still today, Chakra is perceived as science, in that various energies and their source locations in our body reflect universal bio-psychological laws of matter and consciousness.

Diagram of Chakras

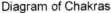

7th Chakra
Calvaria (area at top of head)
Colour: Blue/purple
Endocrine Gland: Pineal Gland
Part of the body that it controls:
Upper part of brain, right eye

5th Chakra
Throat
Colour: Blue
Endocrine Gland: Thyroid Gland
Part of the body that it controls:
Bronchial tube, vocal organs, lungs,
alimentary canal

6th Chakra
Head
Colour
Indigo Blue
Endocrine Gland: Pituitary Gland
Part of the body that it controls:
Lower brain, left eye, ear, nose,
nervous system

4th Chakra
Heart
Colour: Green
Endocrine Gland: Thymus
Part of body that it controls:
Heart, Blood, Vagus Nerve,
Circulatory System

3rd Chakra
Solar Plexus
Colour: Yellow
Endocrine Gland: Pancreas
Part of body that it controls:
Stomach, Liver, Gall Bladder,
and Nervous System

2nd Chakra
Sacrum
Colour: Orange
Endocrine Gland: Sexual Gland
Part of the body that it controls:
Sexual Organs / genitals

1st Chakra
Located between anus and
sexual organs / genitals
Colour: Red
Endocrine Gland: Adrenal Gland
Part of the body that
it controls: Spine, Kidney

Chinese Qi Gong's principles of body and holistic health closely parallel those of Ayurvedic thinking yet afford us a particularly accessible, simple, and practical means of "self help". It is very beneficial to understand the global (and historical) connections of these holistic practices. The more we see the correspondences of ancient Chinese and Indian thought as applied to our health, the richer background we have from which to draw wisdom and guidance. Though fundamental to our lives, there is little formal advice available specifically about applying Qi Gong to diet. This then is mission of this book. However, never loose sight of the connections between all aspects of our health. Fundamentally, to live a healthy and balanced existence, we must breath well, move our bodies, and eat to obtain nature's gift of life to us.

PART 1
QIGONG DIET & BREATH

Qigong is a traditional Chinese method of healthcare with over 3000 years of history. *Qi* means energy in Chinese and, by extension, the energy produced by breathing that keeps us alive; *gong* refers to continual work applied to a discipline or the resultant level of technique. Qigong is both a medical practice and various forms of traditional qigong are also widely taught in conjunction with Chinese martial arts.

Medical Qigong therapy falls into two categories: internal Qi therapy (Qigong practiced by patients) and external Qi (called Wai Qi) therapy. The former refers to Qigong practice by patients themselves to keep fit or to cure their own illnesses, while the latter is the skill used to treat patients by emitting Qi, with the healer situated in a position away from the individual.

The body will be in a state of harmony if vital energy is perpetually flowing smoothly around the body, unhindered, rather like a gentle river. However, if you are stuck inside working in an office building all day long, your head gets tense, and your neck and shoulders stiffen up. Your body becomes lethargic, your legs bloated, and you end up irritated. This is because your body is cut off from its natural world, and is in a state of energy deficiency. At such a point, you stretch, pat yourself down, roll your neck, upon which your head will become clearer and you feel a lot calmer. This amounts to us adjusting our own vital without knowing it, so doing this consciously, and this is what ,gong method is, ameliorating the path of Qi or vital energy.

,e is a plethora of different styles and schools of qigong, each with ,que characteristics. Like meditation there is the quiet practice that ,es not involve moving the body, then the kind that necessitates ,ovement, and the 14 movements that will be introduced in this book fall into the latter category, "movement Qigong".

The Qigong diet is a practical method for creating a new self, where continual effort and re-educating one-self brings the body away from the brink of overheating, to a sensation of healthiness.

The Qigong diet combines nutritional practice with the carrying out of one 35 minute session a day of abdominal breathing exercise. This breathing method has been used as a component of Qigong for over 3000 years by the general population to treat diabetes, hypertension and heart disease. However, it was discovered that this method was also effective for dieting, and has been the subject of research and development at a scientific research facility in Beijing.

Over the last 20 years or so, this method has been used successfully by a great many people, helping them to shed weight.

REGARDING OBESITY

When you consider their diet, it is no wonder that the largest killer of western people is heart disease. It is held that the main causes for this are over-consumption of fast or instant food, and a lack of exercise.

Japan currently enjoys the longest lifespan in the world, but this is attributable to the longevity of those who lived pre-war and during the war, people who ate grain, small fish and subsided on a traditional diet of vegetables, sea food and tofu. However after 1970, the food service industry in Japan took off, bringing in western diets, and because of this the number of Japanese people succumbing to heart disease and colon cancer continues to increase.

An increase in body fat alone means that surplus oxygen and blood are required, resulting in an increased burden on the heart and in fact every organ in the body, heightening the risk of contracting conditions such as heart disease, gallstones, high blood pressure, diabetes, coronary arteries, gout, arthritis and infertility.

WHY WE BECOME OBESE

Eating is something that without doubt encompasses important psychological elements. This is seen commonly in cases where people maintain a healthy diet when in very happy states, but upon facing adversity suddenly relinquish all restraint, and start to binge-eat. Thus people develop excess appetite due to increased stress from work or other sources, relying on the act of eating as a means to feeling good again..

Take Ms. M, who worked in computers and needed to stay up all night at home. One night, finding his stomach rumbling, she cuts herself a piece of cake at one in the morning, and immediately falls into a state of supreme bliss. From then on he makes a habit of eating one big piece of cake every evening, and very soon becomes obese.

A client of mine who teaches at a school in Tokyo despised herself for putting on weight, and wore black clothes so that she might appear just that little bit thinner, she told me. When alone, she was melancholy and felt an insuppressible urge to eat chocolate. She knew it was making her waistline swell, but could not stop. Eating this way would imbue in her a sense of guilt, and although she berated herself for it she just couldn't quit. It was as though she had become addicted to the habit of feeling calm that eating gave her, leading to her obesity.

Consider also that children immersed in the same environment and diet as a parent who is a glutton typically put on weight themselves.

WILL I LOSE WEIGHT THROUGH VIGOROUS EXERCISE?

Taking a look at the ratio of calories burned during aerobics, often considered effective for losing weight, shows that 40 % of calories burned are from body fat, the other 60% coming from sugars. That said, the fact remains that body fat is burned more easily during resting time, when 50% of calories burned are from body fat, and 50% from glucose. This can be easily shown by measuring the quantity of carbon dioxide and oxygen consumed during respiration.

As training intensifies, the consumption of carbon dioxide is exceeded by that of oxygen, and it is sugar rather than body fat that is primarily burned. Because of this, 20-30 minutes pass before body fat ends up being burnt off, leaving one completely exhausted. Contrastingly, the steady practice of Qigong enables one to burn off fat without exerting undue strain on the body. And no matter what kind of diet you are doing, calorie reduction is the main event. Yet where most people go wrong is that the restriction in the amount they eat itself causes stress, upsetting the whole process and thereby ruining the diet. Diet restriction disturbs nutritional balance, leading to a deterioration, rather than improvement, in one's condition. Put simply, a loss of nutritional *balance* slows down basal metabolism, causing a much unwanted weight rebound. But, if one continues the breathing method in the Qigong diet described in this book, one becomes able to exert control over stress and appetite by oneself.

WHY IS THE QIGONG DIET SO EFFECTIVE?

The Qigong diet hinges on abdominal breathing, which involves pushing out the stomach when inhaling, and sucking it in when exhaling. Even taking just one big abdominal breath will show a marked change in the flow of blood in the body.

The heart is perpetually pumping blood around the veins, delivering nutrients to every remote part of the body, with an unrelenting metabolism that sends toxins and waste products to the liver and kidney. Toxins and waste products are then excreted outside of the body. Conscious breathing allows us to artificially add new power to the body. It is held that humans only use one fifth of their lungs in daily life, this stemming from the relationship between humans becoming Homo erectus and the fact that the presence of gravity on earth means that there is a disparity in the amount of blood that flows to the upper and lower parts of the lungs.

Abdominal breathing

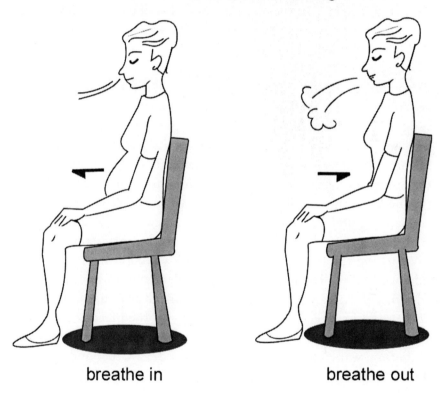

breathe in   breathe out

Loosening the stomach muscles while doing abdominal breathing enables nearly 100% utilization of lungs, and the higher infusion of oxygen leads to a decrease in the number of heartbeats. This increase in oxygen puts more pressure on internal organs and blood vessels makes for the smooth passage of blood flowing into the corner of every capillary, limb and the head. As fresh blood is inexorably linked to the regenerative ability of the skin, one can regain smooth skin, which is resistant to spots, wrinkles and freckles. It amounts to a self-induced internal massage, a naturally remedying posture in the whole body.

Just as in nature, the cosmic dual forces of yin and yang exist in our bodies. As the sun rises and we open our eyes, yang goes into ascendancy filling the body with vitality, activating the internal organs, and the nervous and endocrine systems, and of course the brain. At night, the energy of yin increases and with it its suppressing effect, slowing the metabolism and causing sleepiness. In contemporary biology this natural biorhythm is said to be the reciprocal agitation of parasympathetic and sympathetic nerves. The sympathetic can be seen as an accelerator and the parasympathetic as a brake.

When practicing the breathing method of the Qigong diet, it is possible to render the body into a state somewhere between yin and yang, where neither the sympathetic nor parasympathetic nerves are in a state of ascendancy. Human feelings are passively relaxed, and biologically alpha waves become the predominant brain wave when a state of relaxation is reached. At such a juncture, the part of the body that becomes most active is a place known as the pituitary gland, an endocrine gland where hormones are secreted. The pituitary gland is no bigger than the end of our little finger, but plays a pivotal role in adjusting the workings of the internal secretion instruments inside our bodies. The internal secretion glands have the function of adjusting the release of hormones, which are all awry due to the stress of diet and its attendant eating restrictions. The breathing method allows the release of the hormone melatonin, which eases the stress of dieting; warding off the possibility of a drastic rebound once the diet is over.

Anyone can begin the Qigong diet, but all should be careful of over-slimming. A woman's menstrual cycle could even stop. Health must be prioritized above our external image. Body fat is no enemy either. It is a heat-retainer for the body, stores energy, and is a structural component of the cellular membrane and hormones. We need it, so stop the diet when you have attained a reasonable body weight for yourself.

One way to evaluate ones own weight is by using the Body Mass Index (BMI). BMI is calculated as follows:

$$Body\ Weight \div Height \div Height.$$

To calculate BMI, take the weight (kg) and divide it by height (m).

WEIGHT STATUS

Below 18.5 Underweight
18.5 - 24.9 Normal
25.0 - 29.9 Overweight
30.0 and Above Obese

Keep in mind however that BMI is very general guide and variation in muscle mass will skew the results significantly.

OBJECTIVES OF THE QIGONG DIET BREATHING METHOD

1. Burn off body fat. The source of our energy should be our body fat, as opposed to the food that we consume.

2. Restrict extreme appetite and reduce feeling of being hungry

3. Reduce the mental stress that coincides with dieting

PUTTING THE QIGONG DIET BREATHING METHOD INTO PRACTICE

There are two concurrent exercises of 15 and 20 minutes respectively, to practice daily as follows.

Breathing Exercise Number 1 (15 minute minutes)

Sit on a chair and place cushions and pillows on your knees.

make your left hand into a fist, and wrap your right hand around it

(Men are to have their hands the other way round)

With your elbows pointing out, breathe in slowly through the nose to full capacity.

Placing both elbows on the cushion put your hands against your forehead

Expanding your lower stomach, take a slow deep breath through your nose, and then exhale 70% from your mouth while sucking in your lower stomach, hold your breath for two seconds and then release the remaining 30% by sucking in the whole of your stomach.

Point• With this exercise, please fully focus your consciousness onto your breathing and nothing else.

How your hands should be

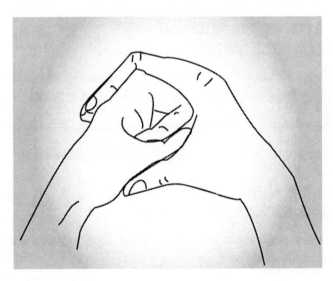

BREATHING METHOD FROM
THE FRONT AND THE SIDE

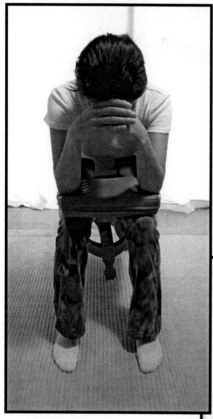

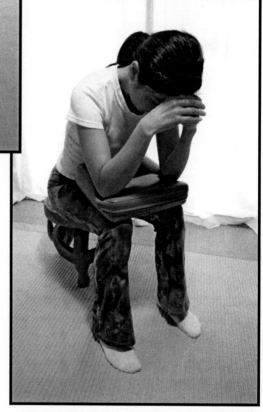

BREATHING EXERCISE NUMBER 2 (20 MINUTES)

Remove the cushions from your knees, lightly close your eyes, and place the back of your right hand on top of the palm of your left, with the two thumbs touching each other.

(Males should have their hands the other way around)

Picture illustrating how your hands should be

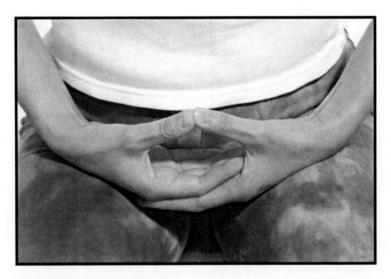

Point: Stick the tip of your tongue onto your upper palate, and slightly raise your jaw.

1) Breath in *slowly* through your nose while expanding the abdomen, and then exhale at normal speed while sucking in the abdomen (5 minutes).

2) Breath in *at regular speed* through your nose while expanding the abdomen, and then exhale from the mouth while sucking in the abdomen (5 minutes).

3) Breath in *slowly* through the nose while expanding the abdomen, breathe out slowly from the mouth while sucking in the abdomen (10 minutes).

Point• With regard to the 20 minute session for *Breathing Exercise 2*, continually envision the image of a burning orange ball, much like the sun, around your abdomen. Try to be vaguely aware of this light while your eyes are closed. It doesn't matter if your eyes are partially open while doing this.

By envisioning this orange ball of light, one recharges virility and strengthens immunity, and amplifies one's desire to live. While practicing, even if unnecessary thoughts and ideas within your mind rise up and interrupt you, hold steady the image of these stray thoughts being sucked into and burned up altogether by the orange ball of light.

Keiko Murakumo

Picture of breathing method for Exercise Number 2
FRONT AND SIDE.

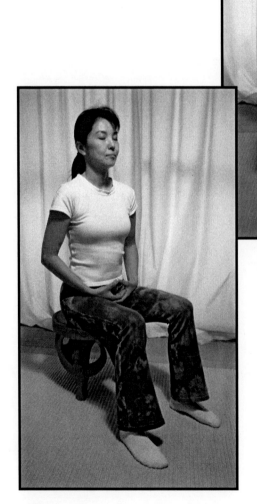

Be sure to carry out Practices Numbers 1 and 2 for 35 minutes every day. The speed at which you lose weight varies from person to person as it depends on the extent of one's body weight, but on average, roughly over a 60 day period one can lose one eighth one one's body weight and in 30 days one tenth. The most ideal time frame for carrying out this practice is before going to sleep, from 11pm to 1am, but two or three hours either side of this won't make much difference.

The Right Environment for Breathing Exercises

While carrying out your breathing exercises, please refrain from leaving the TV on, going to the toilet, answering the phone or breaking off to join your family for dinner. If you do have to leave your session for some reason, you will have to start all over again. Please try and create an environment where you can relax by yourself. You might want to burn some essential oils, or play some calming music perhaps. Try and wear clothes that do not inhibit the free movement of your body.

Due to your parasympathetic nerves becoming dominant (relax mode) during breathing exercises you may become incredibly sleepy, but if you go to sleep the beneficial effects will be lost, so endeavor to stay awake until the end. Your breathing pace should be slow, breathing all the way in deeply and then exhaling completely.

Regarding physical sensations and reactions that may occur during breathing practice

There are various temporary reactions that you may encounter while life energy is in abundance during practice. These include parts of the body warming up or cooling down, a feeling of pins and needles, or maybe excess salivation. These effects coincide with the quashing of pent-up stress, and will pass. Simply continue breathing exercises without paying too much attention to such sensations. Particularly obese people may find that sitting down for a whole 35 minutes induces poor blood flow in certain areas of the body, resulting in pins and needles in your bottom half, and stiffness from the back of the head down to the shoulders. Ease off as much as you are able to, and by mentally willing a sense of calm you can make these sensations abate.

The feeling of finding it hard to take deep breathes manifests when the pace of your spirit and that of your heart are out of sync. Try your utmost to relax, and aim to align and tune the movement of your stomach and breathing with your senses and consciousness.

Changing for the better

Although it depends greatly on the individual, in the same way that picking rubbish and silt from a riverbed will cause the river to flow smoothly again, the process of dieting may well bring out latent wear and tear to a head. For example, lethargy and a light headache are seen as an auto-purificatory reaction that signals a change for the better. Please see this in terms of the body excreting toxins from within.

As the body is purified, such toxins will gradually disappear.

One proviso – refrain from practice if you are receiving treatment at a hospital for an injury, on prescription medicine, have a chronic malady or a particularly weak constitution.

What about getting hungry while I am on the Qi Gong Diet?

It really depends on the person in this case. Although following exactly the same diet, some people are absolutely fine with it and don't complain of hunger, while others are absolutely ravaged with hunger.

There are those of us who are convinced that we can't work unless we eat a lot, that we can't get ourselves going, and as a result cannot tear ourselves away from our hearty eating habits. We fail to lose weight as we are deceived by both ourselves and by the tempting words of others, giving in to snacking between meals, telling ourselves that a little bite here and there won't hurt, or that without something sweet we'll run out of energy .

One client immediately commenced the Qi Gong diet because he had seen many of his own friends who practice it shape up nicely. On coming in to have himself weighed several days later, he immediately got angry with me, saying "I work all day, how on earth can I function properly on this kind of diet! There's no way someone like me with Qids can have time to do the breathing practice!" I reminded the client that I am merely a medium for assisting people to lose weight. On hearing this, he commented "Oh well, in that case I suppose I must persevere and throw myself into it again", but the fact remains that if you don't properly comprehend the Qi Gong diet, you tend to end up blaming your failure to lose weight on other people and the method itself.

The abundance of faddish diets and the wave of product commercials lead people to think they can lose weight in no time. They attempt one new diet after another still thinking they can eat a lot and lose weight in a short time without even doing any exercise. Perseverance and effort is replaced with reliance on supplements and unnatural dieting techniques, leading to weight gain once again, or worse illness. If you truly want to get rid of the reserves of fat that have built up inside you over a long period of time, your own effort and dedication are absolutely essential

SUPPRESSING HUNGER PANGS

Combining the Qi Gong Diet program with the breathing practice can enable you to suppress extreme pangs of hunger, but it does not mean that these pangs will disappear completely. In fact, at the beginning of the diet when you are still getting used to the dieting menu, you may well feel positively gripped by hunger. It depends on the person, but if you feel a bit starved in between meals and find yourself reaching for a snack, just having a glass of water or a cup of tea can diminish the hunger pangs temporarily, but if doing this even a few times a day does not suppress the feeling, try the following breathing technique when you simply cannot bear the hunger any longer.

Breathing Method for Suppressing Hunger During Qi Gong Diet

Place you left hand on your chest, and your right hand over your abdomen.

(Men do the opposite way around)

When inhaling, expand your chest to enable a deep breath

When exhaling expand your abdomen

This counts as one breath, and altogether do between 40-60 breaths to calm you down and relax.

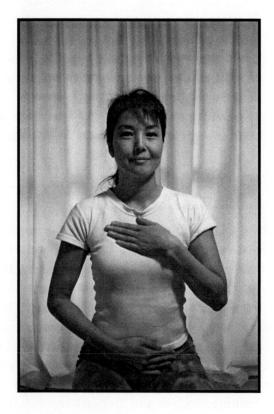

Usually within 3-7 days the body adjusts to the Qi Gong Diet. If you can get over this initial period then the hard work is done. With each day, the burning hunger pangs decrease; one's condition improves, and one starts to feel a sense of ease.

The breathing method loses effectiveness if the time spent on it reduces, so make absolutely sure to stick to 35 minutes. If you wish to dedicate more time than this, then it would be best to add an extra 5-10 minutes onto the second segment of Breathing Method Number 2.

GIVE A LOT OF THOUGHT TO WHAT YOU EAT DURING YOUR DIET

Plain and simple, you can lose weight by reducing the amount you eat, but what we eat each day is our vital source of energy and health maintenance. If one maintains an extreme food-restricted regimen, the body will resort to the glycogen reserves that are stored in the brain, liver and muscles to gain its large supply of energy, and when this has run out it will start to break down the stores of protein in the muscles.

With this, muscles shrink and then a reduction in basic metabolic rate (the amount of energy consumed just for respiration) occurs, meaning that one could actually end up in a situation where it is easy to accumulate fat.

QI (VITAL ENERGY) OF FOOD

Whether you are on a diet or not, it is the food that we consume everyday that gives the body energy, corresponds directly to our health, and so deserves our full attention. Eastern Medicine tells us that food heals an ill body.

Rice is a gift from nature, full of the light from the sun and the rich minerals of the earth. Brown Rice ("genmai") is a natural supplement that contains folic acid, various vitamins such as B1. Japanese Miso is a fermented flavoring that serves both to balance the vitamins within the body, and also functions as an antidote to poisons. Tofu, made from Soya beans, is rich in minerals and reduces cholesterol in the body, and also encourages the secretion of hormones in women. The fat of fish reduces cholesterol and *neutral* fats and is good for the heart and blood vessels, preventing the onset of arteriosclerosis and thrombosis. It also has a substance called DHA, which improves brain functioning. The idea that eating seasonal food is connected to longevity is rooted in the fact that the body contains an element which it needs for adapting to the four seasons. This element as such boosts health through maximizing the particular energy that every type of seasonal food brings, while enhancing the functioning of our organs.

Fruits and Vegetables contain potassium, which wards off the risk that salty foods carry, but also provide us with vegetable fiber, the agent that keeps down the cholesterol level in our blood. Carrots contain β Carotene and this in turn becomes Vitamin A inside the body, which has the effect of activating cells and preventing ageing and cancer. The Vitamin C of the radish prevents wrinkles and spots, and raises our immunity to colds, infections and other diseases.

It should be noted that fruits and vegetables function either to warm up or cool down the body. Examples of foods that cool down the body are banana, pineapple, pear, orange, lemon, melon, eggplant, grapes, tomatoes, cucumber, watermelon, lettuce, white cabbage, mountain potato, clams, crab, squid, curry, coffee, and green tea. These are negative (yin energy) foods, but there are also positive (yang energy) foods which have the opposite effect, warming up the body. Examples of foods that heat up the body are burdock, carrot, lotus root, spring onion, onion, mountain potato, ginger, garlic, shallots, Chinese chives, red-hot chili peppers, prawns, lamb, chicken, beef, liver, cheese, and tea. Furthermore, there are the so-called "neutral foods" that neither heat up nor cool down the body, and these include apples, brown rice, corn, the potato family, Soya beans, cherries, peaches, strawberries, honey, and brown sugar. One should select food that befits his or her physical constitution.

Physical constitutions fall into two types, the yin /negative and yang / positive. People with a yang constitution have a body that is perpetually charged with vigor and warmth, characterized by a rosy, ruddy complexion, but occasionally also shortness of breath, spots or blemishes on the skin, and susceptibility to high blood pressure. Yin/ negative physical constitutions are those with a colder body temperature, and are lacking in vigor and warmth, and in certain nutrients,. These people are often pale, get tired easily and tend towards having low blood pressure. There are also neutral physical constitutions that are neither of these extremes. Yang-types must be careful not to eat foods that cool down the body, and conversely it would be wise for Ying-types to avoid foots that heat up their bodies.

Plants as a single unit are completely balanced, and if eaten raw can provide all the natural vitamins that the body needs. When processed, they lose vitamins and minerals. Eating processed fruits and vegetables with artificial additives and preservatives will lead to nutrient depletion. Vegetable fiber cleanses the insides of the intestines, but processed vegetables lack this vital fiber. Preservatives and artificial additives are not good for the body and so should be avoided. Instead opt for organically-grown foods whenever possible, or at least foods with no pesticides. Watch also your salt intake as too much can lead to blocked circulation and then high blood pressure, strokes, and other conditions that stem from clogged arteries.

During a diet, take pleasure in assembling and preparing the food, and make it look delicious. When you do sit down to eat, it is important to give thanks for what you are about to partake in. Food is a gift from the precious earth.

Suggestions for Meals During the Qi Gong Diet

Whichever way you look at it, the reason that we get fat is because our energy intake is larger than the amount of energy used, so bear this in mind and try to reduce foods you have eaten too much of until now. If you have always gorged yourself on ice cream and cakes, try and cut these out. Break the habit of always having high-calorie desserts, and if you are someone who can put away a whole bag of crisps, or likes to treat yourself to a sweet desert and some fruit after dinner, try and modify your eating patterns. Start by giving up cramming your tea and coffee with sugar and creamy milk, and endeavor to stop filling yourself up with snacks between meals. If you are a beer drinker who likes to chase your drink with some fatty foods every day, try and move away from this habit.

I earnestly recommend a diet based on macrobiotic natural (whole) foods.

Key points regarding what to eat while dieting

I'd like to explain in a little more detail a few tips that are good for keeping calories down during the Qi Gong diet. The basic rule of thumb when dieting is to stop short of stuffing oneself, exercising moderation every mealtime. After putting something in your stomach, it takes about 20 minutes for this message to be delivered to the brain, so the feeling of being full and satisfied comes 20 minutes after you have finished eating. Needless to say if we eat until we are completely full up every meal-time, we end up taking in 20% in excess of our capacity every time we eat. And when this happens, our stomach expands a little to accommodate the excess of food, and the next mealtime we have to eat even more to fill this growing stomach if we are to feel satiated, making it very difficult to lose weight. So, when dieting, eat an amount which is just short of "enough", taking plenty of time to eat it.

As was previously mentioned, the things that we need to rule out when dieting are foods that are high in saturated fat and processed sugar content (especially high calories). This is not just for the sake of losing weight, but is all about doing the right thing for our *health*. Reducing the amount of calories we take in reduces by-products of food, which in turn reduces the amount of reactive oxygen that is released into our bodies, preventing the early onset of ageing. Reactive oxygen is the main element in free radicals which are the main cause of damage to other cells in the body and resultant ageing.

When eating out in a restaurant, choose either fish that is low in fat or choose chicken, and ask the person in charge to have the chef cook it without using butter or margarine, instead steaming it or cooking it in the oven. Avoid fried foods at all costs. In place of the potatoes and rice that come with your main course, opt instead for broccoli, carrots and other vegetables, and don't feel the need to eat every single thing that is served up on your plate, leaving some or taking it home with you.

When ordering a salad, ask the waiter to bring the sauce or dressing separately, and remember to lower the amount of dressing you put on your salad. If you are eating fast food, don't opt for hamburgers which are high in fat and covered in sauce, instead go for chicken burgers without sauce and mayonnaise, and eat plenty of salad with it, leaving half of the bread. Avoid sour cream and cheese.

The actual making of bread involves a lot of butter, margarine and shortening agents.

In the case of donuts and pastries, a large amount of sugar, milk and oil is used so if you are on a diet these are foods that you should definitely not be eating.

Juices, carbonated drinks and supplement-type drinks are usually ingested straight from the refrigerator and as they are cold, so one cannot taste how sweet they really are. They actually contain a lot more sugar than you might think. When it comes to coffee, some dieters think that they are doing themselves a favor by not adding sugar and just a small cup of cream, but this cream actually contains twice as many calories as sugar, so don't forget that these little everyday habits that we take for granted are actually another cause of obesity. When on a diet, as much as possible drink mineral water and tea minus the sugar and milk.

Eating out generally leads to an excess intake of calories, so as far as possible opt for a lunch box of vegetables and low-fat cheese / cottage cheese, or whole-wheat sandwiches containing hummus or something similar, whole-wheat pasta, vegetable burritos, accompanied by picked vegetables.

When you are cooking for yourself at home, using mustard and other spices in your recipes enables you to get away with eating a smaller amount, and when you are slicing vegetables or making soup remember that large slices of vegetables take longer to chew and this enables you to feel full up while having eaten less. When shopping always scrutinize the labels of the product and be aware of the flavorings and the kind of oil that they contain, watching out for how many calories the package contains. Cut right down on refined products, and make a point of selecting foods which enter the blood stream slowly, and are absorbed and digested slowly, such as whole-wheat pasta, brown rice, whole-wheat bread, beans, and vegetables.

One thing that makes losing weight easier is to drink 1.5-2 liters of water everyday on an empty stomach. This is because in order for the stomach to metabolize the water, the kidneys require a large amount of energy which in turn raises the metabolism, and consequently burns off a lot of calories. Try and find time to drink water during breaks at work and before meals. Drinking a large amount of water while eating itself causes indigestion and blood sugar levels to rise, and in turn induces insulin, causing a considerable impediment to your diet.

Insulin is a hormone that emanates from the pancreas and changes glucose into energy, storing it in the cells. Regulating blood sugar levels and conserving energy, it is absolutely indispensable. Our fat cells are controlled by insulin. If there is insulin in the blood stream, neutral fats are assiduously created and stored in the body, but conversely if insulin is lacking then neutral fats will be broken down and released as a source of energy.

When dieting, stop eating in-between meals and if you do feel peckish during the day, drink lots of mineral water or tea, and if this doesn't keep a rumbling stomach at bay, refer to the preceding paragraph about how to carry out breathing practices which are effective in warding off hunger pangs.

Within human beings is a cycle whereby absorption inhibits excretion. From the time you rise in the morning until about midday, a hormone called motilin is released from the gastric lining. Motilin is a hormone which effectively functions to cleanse the inside of the intestines and when it is working well we are able to produce excreta. However if we put food in our stomachs, it is difficult for motilin to be released and excreta remains in the intestines, obstructing the purification and cleansing of our bodies, so bearing this in mind, try to cut out breakfast altogether or keep what you eat first thing to a minimum and take a liquid diet in order to reduce the burden placed upon the stomach.

Carbohydrates that are highly prevalent in the starch of grains, potatoes, vegetables, beans and pulses are digested inside the body and broken down into glucose, and on being absorbed into the small intestine, enter the blood stream and are incorporated into cells as a source of energy.

Carbohydrates take the form of glucose, known also as blood sugar, and directly deliver fuel to the central nervous system, brain and muscles. Not all carbohydrate foods are created equal, some are absorbed and digested quickly, and others slowly. The glycemic index or GI describes this difference by ranking carbohydrates according to their effect on our blood glucose levels. After ingesting carbohydrates which are digested and absorbed quickly, the speed at which they are turned into glucose is also fast and thus enter the blood stream very rapidly. On the other hand, carbohydrates which are digested and absorbed slowly, after being ingested, become glucose very slowly and thus their entrance into the blood stream is, by the same token, slow.

I touched on this previously, but the level of sugar in the bloodstream is regulated by insulin, produced in the pancreas. Eating processed foods which do not contain dietary fiber and which are quickly digested and absorbed, such as bread and cookies made with wheat flour, sweets, cakes, carbonated drinks, juices made from concentrate, jam, potato chips, white rice, causes a large amount of insulin to be unnecessarily secreted. Some of this insulin is used in muscles but the excess blood sugar that remains all becomes neutral fat. If you continue to eat these kinds of food for a long time and overwork your pancreas, you risk not only obesity and coronary diseases, but also hyperlipidaemia (excessive fat in blood), high blood pressure, diabetes, and progressive hardening of the arteries leading to arteriosclerosis. At which point a vicious circle occurs whereby the large amount of insulin being secreted leads the blood sugar level to drastically drop, and one feels hungry soon after eating and wants to eat more. However if one stays away from such carbohydrates, and can instead consume carbohydrates which are low on the GI index, there is nothing to worry about.

Unrefined, low GI carbohydrates contain dietary fiber, whose composition also includes protein, and most of the vitamins and minerals and antioxidants needed to fight off illnesses. Compared to fat and protein, such carbohydrates are the premium and preferable fuel for the body.

For example, if one eats all-grain cereals, brown rice, or all-grain bread and pasta, beans / pulses, sweet potatoes and other vegetables, all of which fall into the category of non-refined carbohydrates, the amount of glucose that enters the bloodstream is minimal so the pancreas is not heavily burdened and your blood sugar level does not experience drastic fluctuations. Over a period of time, this kind of carbohydrate maintains the right level of blood sugar so one does not encounter a feeling of hunger after eating. The above-mentioned foods leave you feeling full after eating them, and require a lot of chewing so it takes time to eat them and one can manage to feel satisfied eating less. Less body fat is accrued, and to top it all off, they provide ideal fuel for the body. These sorts of carbohydrates, thus, are on the side of the dieter.

Actually, irrespective of whether they come from carbohydrate, protein or fat, excessive calories all turn into fat in the end, and especially calories that come from a high intake of fat. It is well-founded that eating too much protein such as the kind found in meat can lead to kidney stones, osteoporosis, high-blood pressure, and the ageing of arteries. This is because when protein in meat is metabolized, it turns into harmful amino acids and when these are used in the muscles and other organs, harmful by-products of proteins such as uric acid and ammonia are produced, which are bad for the body. Such toxins eat away at our bodies. A case in point is that in Japan, one does not see many cases of obesity and coronary disease among elderly people who have a high-carbohydrate diet, yet in the West where young people have a high intake of fat and protein, there are increasingly a large number of cases of diabetes and obesity being documented. So, there is no need to eat meat every mealtime as it is perfectly sufficient to have one high-quality protein meal a day, possibly some beans / pulses, fish, cheese or nuts.

Is it not the case that cows and horses only eat the grass that grows beneath them yet they have supple and strong bodies?

What about drinking alcohol when on a diet? Well, alcohol is usually broken down inside the body and becomes carbon dioxide and water. During this process it does release energy, but this is consumed while one is in a state of inebriation so the alcohol itself does not necessarily directly lead to obesity, but the whole thing about getting fat through drinking has to do with the kind of food people tend to eat while they are consuming alcohol. As the energy intake from alcohol is used up before anything else, the food that we eat while drinking is not effectively used, and instead turns to fat and is stored in the body. In other words, when we eat high-calorie snacks and finger food while we drink, they remain in the body for a long time and the digestion is put off until later, meaning we get fatter. Another thing about alcohol is that it can exacerbate the appetite and this can interfere with the metabolism of minerals in the body, so one has to really watch what one eats when having a drink. Skipping your main meal and just drinking is another bad move as not only does it mean that our calorie intake will be out of kilter, but will also put a strain on both the stomach and the liver. So. Don't eat fried food or snacks and sweets, and instead opt for low calorie snacks that have been made with green and yellow vegetables or beans, making sure that your intake of minerals is balanced. Drinking alcohol on an empty stomach means that it is very easy to get drunk, and our attitude towards dieting is weakened and we are easily tempted to eat the wrong kinds of foods, so care needs to be exercised. Drink a glass of water before indulging in alcohol, and try to stay awake for three hours after you have finished drinking. Whether on a diet or not, alcohol is something to be enjoyed only in moderation.

One final point I would like to make is that we should not rely solely on food from outside for energy, and remember that carrying out 35 minutes of breathing exercises a day will serve to release energy that is stored in fat in our bodies. Our inner organs are active while we sleep. What provides this energy are the stores of fat that are retained inside of us. The most ideal time to carry out breathing exercises is at night, because it is then that our parasympathetic nerve is in the ascendancy. It is at this time that we can raise breathing exercises to their optimum in burning fat. Going to sleep after carrying out breathing exercises will bring out their maximum potential, so after you have done them it is not wise to stay up late working on the computer or the like.

Bear in mind also that when on the Qi Gong diet it is important to exercise and walk regularly, making sure that your muscle mass does not decreases, and that you get in such shape that you do not rebound to former habits once the diet is finished.

IS YOUR BODY TYPE "YIN" (NEGATIVE) OR "YANG" (POSITIVE) ?

Through eating a diet that is best suited to your body type can play a large part in becoming more healthy.

Have a look at the table below and check which most applies to you.

Is your face shape..	A Long and thin	B Round-face
Color of Face?	A Pallid	B Dark Red
Your body	A Tends to get cold	B Tends to heat up
Height?	A Tall	B Short
What shape is your body in?	A Soft, flabby	B Toned, taut
Palms of your hands?	A Moist	B Dry

Voice?	A Quiet	B Loud
Way of speaking?	A Slow and calm	B Fast and aggressive
Behavior and actions?	A Slow	B Fast
Personality?	A Patient and gentle	B Impatient and restless
Way of thinking?	A Passive, ponderous	B Positive, proactive
Condition in the morning	A Dozy for a while	B Wide awake straight away
White of the eyes are?	A Slightly blue-ish color	B Slightly yellow-ish color
Color of Eyelids ?	A Pale pink	B Red
Eyelids?	A Puffy, swollen	B Not puffy or swollen
Pulse?	A Slow	B Fast
Blood Pressure?	A Low	B High
Body Temperature?	A Low	B High
Appetite?	A Small	B Large
Color of Urine?	A Weak, diluted	B Thick
Color of Faeces?	A Soft and yellowish	B Hard and blackish-brown
Are your hands and feet?	A Cold	B Warm

If you answered mainly "A", your body tends towards yin (negative) and if mainly "B", yang (positive).

If you had an equal amount of both or neither A nor B applies to you, then your body type can be called "neutral".

	Yin "Negative"	Yang "Positive"
Breakfast	• Carrot and orange juice, or hot unpasteurised Soya milk (with a little cinnamon powder) • Alternatively, Oatmeal • In addition to the above, hot tea, tea with juice from grated ginger, or herb tea • (do not add cream or sugar)	• Unpasturized Soya milk and banana juice • Alternatively low-fat plain yoghurt • Or cold unpasturized Soya milk • In addition to the above, green tea or herb tea • (do not add cream or sugar)
Lunch	• Vegetables • Beans (Tofu is fine) • Whole-grain bread or brown rice ("genmai) Or whole-grain spaghetti • Fish or meat (with no fat on it) or non-fat cheese, nuts of some variety	• Vegetables • Beans (Tofu is fine) • Whole-grain bread or brown rice ("genmai) Or whole-grain spaghetti • Fish, Chicken (skinless) or non-fat cheese, nuts of some variety
Dinner	• Vegetables • Beans (Tofu is fine) • Whole-grain bread or brown rice ("genmai) • Fish or meat (with no fat on it) • Seaweed of some kind	• Vegetables • Beans (Tofu is fine) • Fish or Chicken (skinless) • Seaweed of some kind

Forbidden Foods: Snacking in between meals, fruits / vegetable juices not on the menu, soft drinks, sweets, bread and bread crutons, foods containing refined white flour, milk, butter, margarine, lard, beef fat, cream, bouillon etc containing animal fats, white sugar

- If cooking with oil use Canola, Olive or Chestnut oil

- For flavorings, use natural salt or soy sauce, miso, fat-free soup stocks, sauces, or spices. Always make salad dressing yourself. Don't make any fried foods at all.

- When it comes to vegetables, don't just stick to one variety, but eat fungi, root vegetables and seasonal vegetables, all sorts in equal measure.

- Fish, meat, chicken, low-fat cheese, nuts of some variety, should only be eaten once a day (in the above menu these appear in both lunch and dinner, but if you have one of these protein sources for lunch, don't eat it for dinner, and vice versa)

- Drink 1500cc-2000cc per day of water or tea (but not during mealtimes)

- Don't sleep within 3 hours of eating

- Yin "negative" types should add slightly more salt to their food and should try to eat food warm, boiled food that has been cooked for a relatively long time. In particular your evening meal should not contain raw vegetables. When drinking water try to drink hot tea or warm water. At any rate, avoid anything cold before going to bed.

- Yang "positive" types should avoid salty and oily foods as much as possible, and should aim to have a diet centered around raw vegetables that have only been cooked for a minimal amount of time. For flavoring, go for something light, with a dash of vinegar maybe.

- So-called "neutral" types can select either menu.

HOW TO MAKE DELICIOUS BROWN RICE ("GENMAI")

Brown rice is analeptic, health-boosting and as a sprouting living food is jam-packed full of natural vitamins B1, E, minerals and dietary fiber, in every grain. Brown rice has antioxidant properties and prevents the absorption into the body of foreign substances such as pesticides and radiation.

* Cooking Brown Rice ("genmai") in a Thick Stainless Pot

1. Place two cups of brown rice (genmai) in a bowl, pour on water and wash rice. Drain the water out of the bowl and repeat previous steps, adding water again and washing, twice or three times. (finally separating the washed rice with a sieve)

2. Pour water into the stainless pot (1.5-1.8 times amount of rice) and then put the rice you drained in the sieve into the pot. Put the lid on and leave for 2-6 hours.

3. Add a pinch of salt to the pot and turn on the heat. Use a low heat and cook for at least thirty minutes, and then take the heat off. Leave for ten minutes, and it's ready ! Using a wooden spoon or fish slice, turn the rice from top to bottom and mix it around.

*Cooking brown rice in a pressure cooker

Follow the steps above for (1). Add water at a ratio of 1.3-1.5 x water compared to rice, and a pinch of salt, into the pressure cooker. Once the pressure builds up, turn down heat and cook for 20 minutes. Take off the heat and leave until the pressure naturally abates. Using a wooden spoon / fish slice, stir the rice from top to bottom and mix it around without crushing it, and then it is ready.

If you do not eat the brown rice immediately after cooking it, divide it into small portions and get rid of any air, and wrap it as flat and even as possible, either in polythene bags or airtight containers. Once it has cooled down store it in the refrigerator. When eating it, heat it up in the microwave leaving without removing the wrapping. Yang (negative) body types should aim to keep the amount of water added down, making harder rice, and Ying (positive) types should add in extra water aiming for a softer rice. Either way, be sure to chew the rice thoroughly before swallowing.

In order to provide yourself with vitamins and minerals that brown rice cannot provide alone, or if the taste of brown rice is not enough for you, try the following:

Sesame salt version
5 Table Spoons of Black Sesame
1 Tea Spoon of natural salt
Thoroughly mix and stir in the above ingredients.

Japanese-style version
1 Table Spoon White Sesame
1 cup finely grated bonito flakes (available in supermarkets)
50g Cress (finely sliced)
1 Table Spoon Soy Sauce
Splash of Canola Oil

1. Pour the oil into a frying pan, add the cress and stir-fry

2. Add the sesame and mix in well

3. Add the bonito flakes and soy sauce and stir-fry till ready.

Having actually succeeded in getting your weight down, the biggest challenge still lies ahead – the challenge of maintaining your new weight. There is a tendency to suddenly start eating high calorie foods after slimming down, and piling fat back on in the process. Here are some steps to help you exercise control over your weight on a daily basis:

Weigh yourself every morning after bowel movements and passing urine. Know your weight. If it goes up, try to eat less on that day

- To stay in good health, carry out Qi Gong diet breathing exercise no.3 for 15 minutes, at least three times a week

- Be careful not to lose body muscle. Attempt to increase the amount of muscle you have.

- Drink a lot of water outside of meal-times

- Make your evening meal the lightest of the day, and as much as possible avoid eating dessert, fruits, snacks / sweets, instant foods, and manufactured goods containing white sugar and wheat flour. Take care on a daily basis to not consume too much animal fat.
- When eating, always keep balance in mind and create a menu that provides a balance of nutriments.
- Never eat sweet foods on an empty stomach
- If you do end up eating a lot in the evening, refrain from breakfast the next morning (fast for half a day)

WHAT TO EAT AFTER COMPLETING THE DIET

Persevere with the dietary regimen and the breathing practices for one to three months at the outset, and you should end the diet at the point when you reach your own desired weight, but you can make yourself ill by suddenly increasing the amount you eat. To ensure that you don't rebound, for a week after you have finished the diet you should only slightly increase the amount of food in your menu. Secondly, choose ingredients based on how digestible they are, and warm food up before you serve it. Eat easily absorbable foods and your staple should be something soft like rice porridge. The most important point to remember is that in order to stop yourself piling on the pounds again, personal weight control is vital on a daily level, accompanied with measures to build a strong physical frame, such as walking, stretching, doing Qi Gong, Yoga and Meditation.

KEEPING A QI GONG DIET DIARY

What will surely be on your mind just before undertaking the Qi Gong Diet is the creeping doubt about whether you will really manage to follow the regimen and do the breathing exercises for 35 minutes, each and every day.

And this is it. You can do it if you really want to. If you find yourself getting all weighed down by it, or start to succumb to the temptation of instant gratification food, just tell yourself this; "I can do this!"

It is advisable to keep a record of your diet progress. Decide on a period of time in line with your own particular goal, and try to write in it every day. You will include your weight, your thoughts on how the breathing exercises are going, what you have been eating, and also record in detail your feelings on the whole process.

BE BEAUTIFULLY RE-BORN THROUGH THE QI GONG DIET!

You see a profound change in people when they complete the diet. Apart from significant weight loss, they seem to have been in some way reborn. Thanks to new equilibrium in the autonomic nerves one experiences a sense of calm. A better complexion is visible, with the amount of waste products in the body reduced. Skin rejuvenates resulting in the Qi Gong dieter looking younger than their actual age. Wrinkles between the eyebrows fade.   Above all is the sense of accomplishment from having worked hard towards a goal and having succeeded in losing weight. This confidence shines through and is visible in the face. Depending on the individual, symptoms of various conditions are alleviated, including headaches, menstrual pain and irregular periods, backache and high blood pressure, many others.

READ THE SIGNS THAT YOUR BODY OFFERS

Irrespective of diet, practicing Qi Gong heightens sensory awareness. Through Qi Gong we become very sensitive to any slight change in our condition. Some people work hard year after year without taking any holidays, and never seem to catch so much as a cold. They seem to be the very picture of health, but it is these people who may wind up contracting a serious illness. Equally, those who are sensitive to any slight fluctuation in their body and react to it by succumbing to illness every now and then are less likely to contract a serious illness out of the blue. All illnesses, no matter how small, should be viewed in terms of a message from the body that enables you to realign yourself with your health. We would all do well to pay attention to these signs that our body gives us.

DON'T GIVE UP, WHATEVER HAPPENS

Apparently human genes are programmed in a way that allows us to live to 90-120 years without getting ill. We are the architects of the factors that contribute to our illnesses, but we are also born with the ability to heal ourselves. Qi Gong is fantastically effective in maximizing our ability to use this power. Each person has a different level of health and a different history when it comes to illness, so the time it takes to heal varies greatly from person to person. What is important is to persist in self-training, with the conviction that if you strive for something from the bottom of your heart, it can come true.

TESTIMONIES FROM PRACTITIONERS IN JAPAN WHO HAVE UNDERGONE THE QI GONG DIET

Mr. S, Business Executive

"I had wanted to lose weight for ages, but just couldn't manage it. On some occasions I embarked on a diet only to find myself actually gaining weight. As I approached 50 I felt that it couldn't go on any longer, and when I heard about the Qi Gong diet it struck me as the ideal weight-loss method and started it straight away. What I noticed primarily was that the quantity of food I had got used to up till now had considerably decreased. I didn't feel gripped by hunger, and actually appreciated how delicious vegetables were. It also dawned on me that I had been eating un-necessarily and putting extra strain on my body."

Mrs. K, Civil Servant.

"To be quite honest, I didn't hold out much hope at the beginning but I made a promise to myself to see it through. The food restriction element left me feeling hungry, and doing the abdominal breath-ing exercises everyday had its tough moments, but I persevered with it. Now I have got where I wanted to, and I do feel that you can do whatever you want if you put your mind to it. My body is now light-er, and my autonomic nerve deficiency has completely cleared up."

Mr. S, Business Owner

"Relying only on western medicine, I was totally stuck in a rut for the last ten years, and I can't think of one day when I wasn't mentally or physically beleaguered. A friend introduced me to the Qi Gong diet and I so I took it up, although half in doubt about its effectiveness. I nearly gave up at one point but somehow I managed to maintain it for the whole 30 days, after which I really did sense a fundamental shift in both my body and mind. I felt that I had been living a lie up until then, looking back on my previous life. Without further ado, I am going to totally apply myself to self-training.

Mr. M, age 70s

"I managed to resist food even when it was put right in front of me and my weight definitely dropped. There were some slightly harsh points where I just couldn't seem to lose any weight, but I kept my chin up and reached my target weight. My body feels liberated, and moving about is just so much easier now, it used to be hell. In winter I used to get rather dry and itchy skin, but thank goodness that has cleared up too. I am going to stay at this weight and really watch what I put in my body."

Mr. K , 40s

"Through doing the Qi Gong diet I felt with my own body just how haphazard and irregular my eating habits have been up until now. Keeping up the breathing exercises and diet regimen to begin with was a tall order, but as each day went on I could definitely feel my body getting lighter. I'm so glad that I did the Qi Gong diet, and I am fully on a health drive from here onwards. Thanks very much"

Y.I, woman

"I'll explain the reason that led to me doing the Qi Gong diet. I turned 36 this year, and happened to have lost my own father when he was the same age. To add to this, my uncle passed away when from a heart muscle blockage four years ago this summer. Last December a teacher at work fell ill from high blood pressure and is still in hospital today. He had internal membrane bleeding. I was suffering from backache and high blood pressure. My starting weight was 96kg, but I managed to get it down to 78kg. Regarding my blood pressure previously was between 150 and 100 at the lowest, at worst between 160-110, but starting the Qi Gong diet brought this down gradually and now it is more like 120-70, and I am maintaining it. What's more, the nauseous feeling that headaches used to bring has disappeared. I can run and walk about with no problems. I use breathing practice to get rid of stress. If I went to the hospital, would I not just be given medicine, and not seen in terms of being a sick person? I am in awe of the way Qi Gong improves things from the very root, contrary to Western medicine. I want to maintain my health and will make sure I don't go putting any weight on again."

Mr. M, School Teacher

"A week into the Qi Gong diet, I got on the scales and found that I had lost 2kg already. The shape of my body was changing somewhat, but the best thing is that my body just feels so much lighter and better. Previously I always felt tired even though I was getting plenty of sleep, but now I am wide awake first thing in the morning and asleep before my head hits the pillow at night."

Mrs. R

"I started the Qi Gong diet because I wanted to do something about the fact that over 40% of my body was composed of fat. I had to take the pressure off my heart by reducing my body weight. 8 years after surgery for uterine cancer, I had a relapse in my lungs. Hearing that losing weight might alleviate my symptoms, I got into the Qi Gong diet. Through following the dietary regimen, the breathing practice, and the lung-improving Kyorin school of Qi Gong that I was taught, I have lost weight little by little. I also stopped coughing up so much phlegm at night. Climbing up the stairs at the station used to leave me wheezing, but my body just feels so much lighter than it used to. I could feel the change in my body, much to my own surprise and delight. The diet left me in such good shape. I sleep a lot more deeply at night, no more coughing up phlegm, and the chest pains I occasionally suffered from have gone away. I have stopped taking all the medicine that I was on for my heart. If you really reach inside, you'll find the answer. I can't thank my teacher enough for the unstinting support and encouragement."

Ms. R, 60s

"For the first 3 days I was hungry the whole time, and inside my head there was this conveyor belt offering cookies and chocolates and sushi going round and round. I was ravenous. Strangely enough then, a week into the diet my stomach got used to it and the pangs disappeared. The whole thing got easier and as the days went on my weight dropped, and I was even enjoying it by then. It made me realize just how excessively I have always eaten up until now. In the end, I lost 11 kg in 2 months. I now want to keep a firm handle on my health."

Ms. Y

"I have tried all sorts of diets and not one of them worked out. To think that you could lose so much weight through a restricted diet and some breathing exercises just never occurred to me. It is certainly a major departure from any knowledge I had on the subject from previous diets. The big lesson for me was realizing the importance of staying in shape in a healthy and correct manner. Measuring exactly what to eat 3 times a day, I gained a new found interest in cooking. It was the breathing method that I owe the most to, though. Early to bed, early to rise, I am now wide-awake when the lights come on, and I just am in such a good condition. I am going to do everything I can to make sure I maintain my current weight."

Ms. U

"Eight years ago I became an insomniac, often feeling lethargic and not even in the mood for eating. I lacked vigor
completely, suffered pins and needles in my feet, bouts of dizziness, my heart beating faster and faster. This went on and on,
an utter nightmare. At the hospital I was told in the internal
medicine department that there was nothing wrong with me
in particular, and was passed onto a different department. I
was prescribed stabilizing drugs for 7 years, but I could not
cure my condition. It was by some act of fate that I heard tell
of the Qi Gong diet, which cured my insomnia and enabled
me to come off the prescription medicine. My head cleared up
tremendously. It really was such a rough period of my life and
I never really felt my true self for ages. I sometimes feel that
this is too good to be true, that I am now able to live a normal
life again."

Mr. M 50s

"I challenged the Qi Gong diet for 30 days At first, I had a ter-
rible headache. On the second day, a constant struggle with the
lure of delicious foods. From the third day onward, I felt light in
a way that I have not for years, and even got rid of my shoulder
tension. It was a total lesson in the importance of improving your
physique through your eating habits, and also how wonderful the
breathing practice is. Rather than the amount of food you actually eat though, it is really the breathing exercises that make you
shed weight the following day. What struck me was how decadent
our eating habits have become, as we can easily subsist on a simple
diet. It is just so bad for our diet to eat so extravagantly. I have
always gorged myself on food with lots of flavoring and various ingredients, so to start with I had a tough time with the diet. I made
the best of it though, and appreciated how nice the simple taste of
lightly cooked vegetables is. In fact, I think I have got my erstwhile
senses of taste and smell back. My weight definitely dropped and I
also see the experience in terms of some decent character building.

I thought about quitting several times in the first week I felt absolutely awful. I've got a taste for some new vegetables now though, and eating a somewhat restricted diet is no longer a chore for me. The breathing exercises were not at all easy for me. I yawned and even wept at some points. My face has a fresh shape to it now, and surprisingly even my tense shoulders and headaches have improved. I have also stopped taking my medicine.

"For the last several years my weight has gradually increased, and a diet alone has not been enough to help me lose any weight. For as long as I can remember I have lived a very unregimented lifestyle, so it wasn't at all easy to change this. It was marvelous that I managed to lose 9kg within just two months of starting the Qi Gong diet. The weird thing was that it didn't feel like such a huge effort, and I never suffered from hunger particularly. I believe that dieting is the first step towards better health, so I am planning to carry on with the Qi Gong from now on."

Ms. K.M

"I turned 50 recently, and without realizing it I got fatter and fatter and before I knew it my weight had reached 62 kg. I was not sure that I would be able to commit to 35 minutes a day of breathing exercises, but with a bit of quiet music on in the background I managed them fine. I was astonished to lose some 2 kg in the first 4 days! In the end my weight dropped 10kg in 2 months. My body fat rate went from 26% to 19 %! Qi Gong has helped me to feel better, and from the outside I look 10 years younger now, which is great."

Ms. M

"I gave the diet a go for 60 days. The view of dieting and eating that I had up until now has been completely turned on its head. I don't really feel like eating meat anymore, and eating less in the evenings is something that comes quite naturally now.

My fiancé remarked on how amazing it was that I lost weight without really stressing out. I can wear a lot of my wardrobe again, my period pains have got better; so many good things have come about because of the diet. I can't wait for my wedding, because everyone will see the new slim me."

Ms. R, 20s

"I've never had any luck with dieting so was somewhat skeptical about this one. I'm really glad that I did it though, as after beginning the Qi Gong diet I started to enjoy exercise more, and re-discovered the taste and smell of vegetables that I had lost for ages. The breathing exercises and restricted diet were not so painful either. The best thing of all though is that a month after starting the diet I became pregnant. I have been unable to get pregnant for ages and it was really worrying me, so I am literally over the moon about it"

PART 2
MOVEMENT

Generally, when people get ill they tend to see themselves in terms of being the victim of an illness. In Chinese medicine, however, if your life energy is out of balance it is attributed to the operation of your mind. If any of the 7 emotions (joy, anger, sorrow, thought, sadness, fear, astonishment) become too extreme, they have a negative influence on the life energy within your body, and this is what becoming ill is defined as.

Put simply, negative thoughts influence the whole body, jeopardizing the workings of the pressure points, impeding the *flow* of the meridians and ultimately damaging the internal organs. This manifests as illness. Over a short period of time, the body can regain its original form, but when stress and tiredness start to be prevalent in the long term, that damage accumulates and can then lead into varying kinds of adult illnesses.

NEGATIVE ENERGY
INVADING THE BODY

Negative emotional energy invades the body through the points on the bottom of the foot, into the meridians

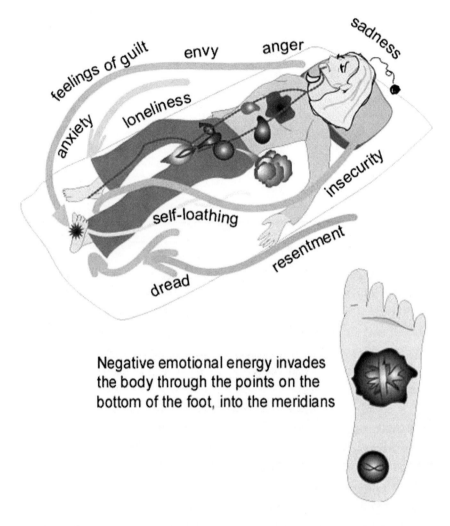

feelings of guilt   envy   anger   sadness

anxiety   loneliness

insecurity

self-loathing

resentment

dread

Negative emotional energy invades
the body through the points on the
bottom of the foot, into the meridians

With today's lifestyles of unbalanced diets and various negative
environmental factors, stagnation of our life energy and dampening
of our internal awareness can easily occur, leading to various health
problems. People are seldom sufficiently attuned to the body and
its constant subtle sensory messages, so that though while they may
have indications of cancer or kidney trouble they cannot detect or
acknowledge any affliction until serious symptoms appear and treatment
becomes far more problematic. It is not just the energy system, but also
the secondary nervous system that is inoperative, and cannot inform
you that you are truly ill. No matter how small symptoms or signals

may seem to be, they are all deviations from your healthiest condition and need to be acknowledged. Thus, whenever such deviations occur, instead of waiting until a genuine named illness requiring treatment occurs, you can take corrective action. One form of such action is to build Qi Gong into your life.

THE EFFECTS OF QI GONG

Immunology is about raising the immune capacity, and in essence tells us that in order to stop ourselves from getting ill, we should aim to calm down agitated nerves, and to focus on relaxing ourselves. Carrying out the 14 Qi Gong movements can lead the body to such a state of relaxation, creating a smoother flow of life energy. Practicing the breathing exercises correctly regulates the balance of the autonomic nerves, breathing life into the functioning of the internal organs.

Through focusing our consciousness, we can render our cerebral cortex into a state of rest. By giving vigor to the brain functions that govern human activity, the brain stem and the interbrain (or diencephalon) our immunity and natural healing ability are also raised.

THE 14 QI GONG MOVEMENTS

GOALS AND BENEFITS

Each of the 14 separate movements has its own name These movements can be adapted to your own particular physical condition. ☒

By moving your body, you stimulate the pressure points, raising the flow of life energy through the meridians, releasing negative energy that your body should expel. You will then harness positive life energy, and in doing so boost the functioning of each internal organ.

DON'T TRY AND RUSH RESULTS, THEY WILL COME.

When practicing, as much as possible try and relax yourself completely. It's really essential to be as calm as you can. In the same way that hasty farming does not enable you to bring the harvest round any quicker, any kind of change that occurs in you will happen over extended time. It is essential to remember that it is the very process of continual rather than intermittent practice that nourishes growth and change. However, if the thought of practice leads you to feel stressed, or you simply cannot find the right time, take a break and return when you are ready and eager rather than forcing it on yourself. The most effective way to gain self-discipline is to shun a sense of misery and stoicism towards your practice while always seeking a positive and enjoyable attitude to practice in.

WHAT ARE THE MAIN POINTS TO BEAR IN MIND WHILE PRACTICING?

Frame of mind - resolve to conquer your ailments and problems.

Clothing —loose and easy, with nothing tight or body hugging.

Food - Avoid practicing when you are full or really hungry.

Place – Find somewhere quiet, with both the appropriate temperature and humidity.

Mindset - Don't practice when your emotions are in a state of turmoil. Do take every opportunity to practice when you are in a positive or pleasant mood

Each movement should be practiced several times, over and over again, slowly going through each and every action, ideally for 15-30 minute periods each time.

It would be fantastic if you can incorporate sessions into your everyday routine, just as you wash your face every morning, but even if you only manage once or twice a week you will begin to see changes in your body as time goes by.

POINTS TO REMEMBER DURING PRACTICE SESSIONS.

1. As you move, be mindful to release any unnecessary power held in your body .

2. practice each Movement about 1 minute each, for a total approximate session time of 15 minutes, as frequently per week as you can, 1 or 2 times at first, increasing to daily sessions.

2. Move very slowly and fluidly, breathing at a calm and steady pace.

3. Hold an image in your mind of yourself consciously drawing life energy from the universe as you work through the session

It is important to note that that the following 14 movements correspond to the 14 bodily Meridians identified by Qi Gong science.

NAMES OF EACH MOVEMENT AND BENEFIT

Number 1. Turning the ball of light (Connecting the Small Intestine Meridian)

Small Intestine Meridian: Is a pair with the heart meridian, and regulates the small intestine.

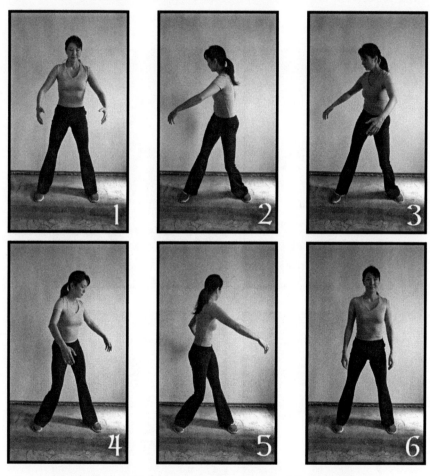

1. Both palms should face each other, as if holding a ball
2. Bend one knee, and twist body as if still holding a ball
3. Bring body back slowly to original position
4. Repeat step 2 in the opposite direction
5. Re-adopt standing position as in step 6
6. Stand straight, with fingers pointed downward, legs slightly apart.

NUMBER 2. DRAWING A RAINBOW WITH YOUR BODY MOVEMENT (CONNECTING THE LUNG MERIDIAN).

Lung Meridian: This route regulates the lungs

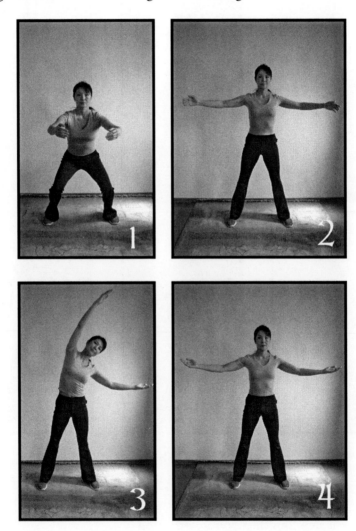

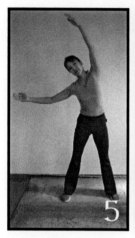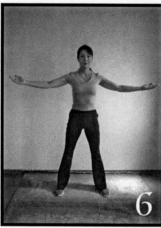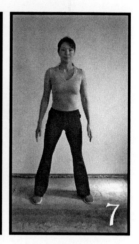

1. Bend both knees and lower hips, extend both arms forward.
2. Straighten legs, and extend both arms out to the side.
3. Raise one arm, tilting slightly to one side
4. Bring arms down
5. Repeat step 3, in the opposite direction
6. Bring arms down
7. Bring both arms down

Number 3. Swimming through clouds (Connecting the Large Intestine Meridian)

Large Intestine Meridian: This is linked to the lung meridian as the two are pairs. This route regulates the functioning of the large intestine.

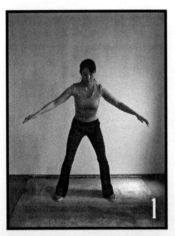
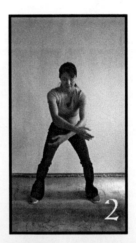
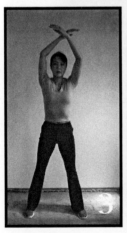
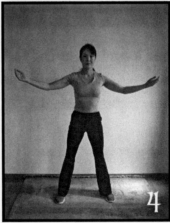
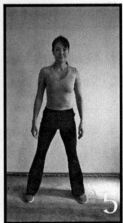

1. Bring arms slowly towards each other
2. Arms cross in front of body, while bending knees
3. While straightening legs, raise arms above head
4. Bring both arms down slowly
5. Revert to standing straight position

Number 4. Letting a small moon out through a window (Connecting the Stomach Meridian)

Stomach Meridian: This route regulates the stomach, taking charge of digestion and absorption.

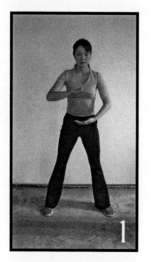
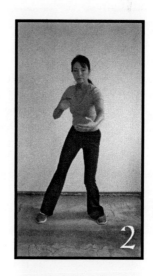
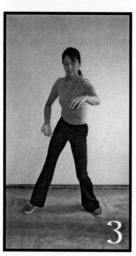
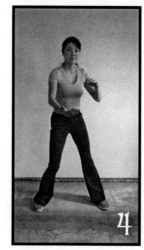

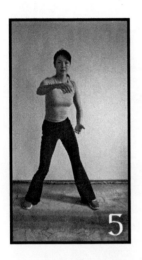 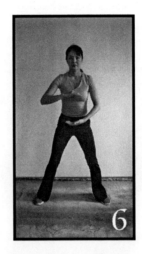 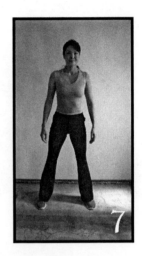

1. Palms face each other, as if holding a ball
2. While bending one knee, slowly extend one arm.
3. Bring extended arm back towards body, with palms facing downwards.
4. Repeat step 2, with opposite arm
5. Repeat step 3, with opposite arm.
6. Re-adopt standing position as in step 1
7. Stand straight; fingers pointed downwards, legs slightly apart.

Number 5. Rowing a boat on the lake (Connecting the Spleen Meridian)

Spleen Meridian: This and the stomach meridian are pairs, and this route is also in charge of digestion and absorption,

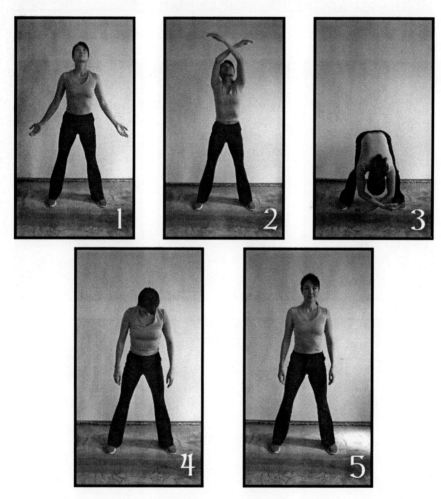

1. Raise both arms up, palms facing upwards
2. Link arms above head
3. Bend over, loosening hips, keeping arms crossed
4. Slowly bring body back to original standing position.
5. Stand straight.

Number 6. Letting up a balloon (Connecting the Heart Meridian)

Heart Meridian: This is the route that regulates the brain and the heart.

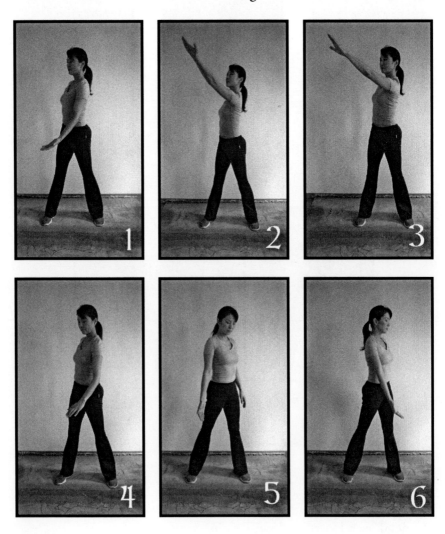

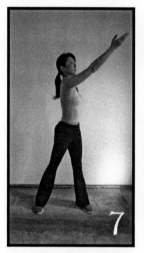 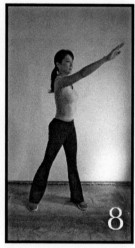 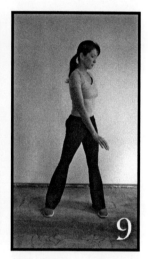

1. Twist body and raise one arm, palms facing upwards.
2. Continue to raise arm
3. Twist palms to face downwards, bring one arm down.
4. Continue to bring arm down
5. Repeat step 1 with opposite arm
6. Continue to slowly raise arm.
7. Raise arm up above head
8. Twist palm to face downwards, bring arm down.
9. Bring arm all the way down.

Number 7. Twisting your upper body to view a distant full moon (Connecting the Heart Meridian)

This is the route that regulates the brain and the heart.

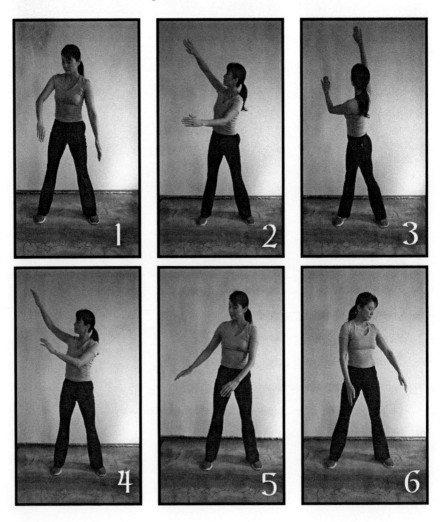

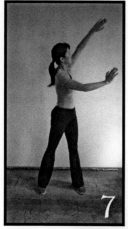
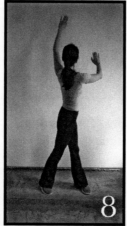
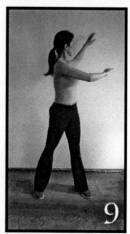

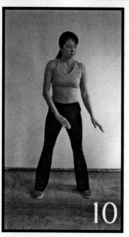
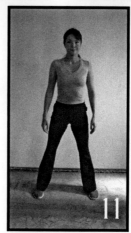

1. While twisting trunk of your body, slowly raise arms
2. Slowly extend arms upwards further, looking over your shoulder. Feet should face forwards, and you are gazing at a faraway sky,
3. Extend arms fully, continuing to twist body, feet facing forwards.
4. Slowly return arms to original position
5. Continue slowly returning arms to original position
6. Repeat step 1, the other way around
7. Repeat step2 , the other way around.
8. Repeat step 3
9. Slowly return arms to original position
10. Bring arms down, towards standing position
11. Stand straight.

Number 8. Creating clouds with both hands (Connecting the Bladder Meridian)

Bladder Meridian: Aside from regulating the bladder, this route also aids in reproduction and ageing.

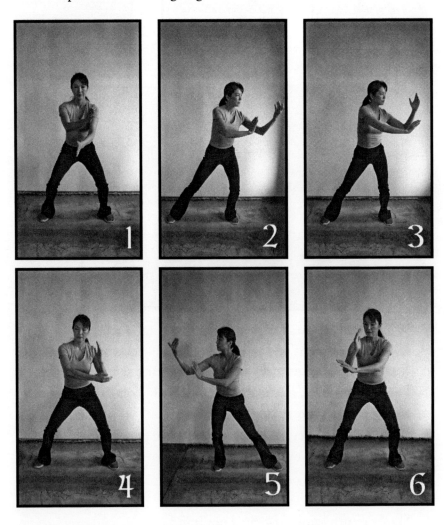

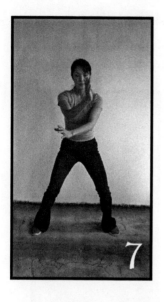 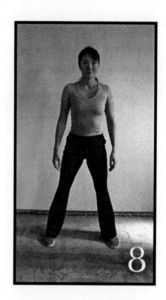

1. With palms facing outwards, bring wrists towards each other, crossing in front of the body.

2. Assume standing position

3. Keeping wrists in this position, squat and lower hips.

4. Keeping hips at the same height, move wrists to one side, making a horizontal movement with you body.

5. Bring wrists across to other side of body, the outer wrist crossing over the inner.

6. Keeping knees bent, slowly move arms horizontally to the other side of the chest.

7. Wrists cross in front of chest

8. Adopt standing position

Number 9. Scooping up seawater and releasing it to the sky (Connecting the kidney Meridian)

Kidney Meridian: This is in a pair with the bladder meridian, regulating the kidney but also concerned with reproduction and ageing.

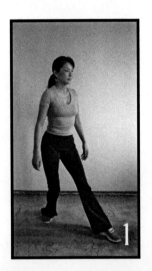
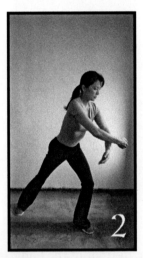

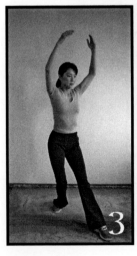
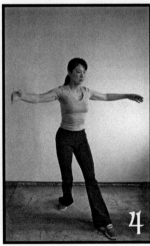
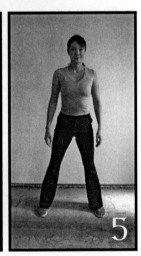

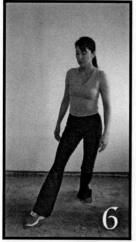
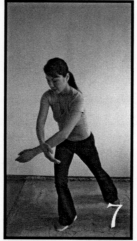
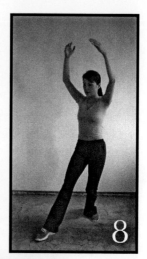

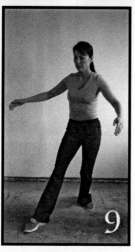
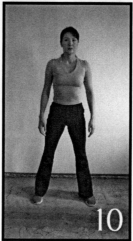

1. With knee bent, extend other leg forward diagonally, keeping it straight.
2. Transfer weight onto front leg, cross wrists in front of body.
3. Raise crossed wrists upwards, slowly transferring body weight onto back leg.
4. Continue to raise wrists above head.
5. Bring both wrists down. Keeping leg out in front.
6. Bring both legs back to standing position,
7. Transfer weight onto front leg, cross wrists in front of body.
8. Raise crossed wrists upwards
9. Bring both wrists down. Keeping leg out in front.
10.Adopt original standing position.

Number 10. The coming and going of waves (Connecting the Heart Meridian)

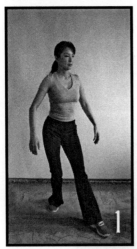
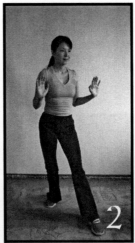
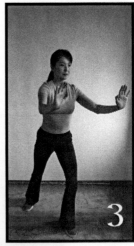
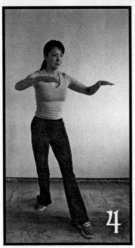
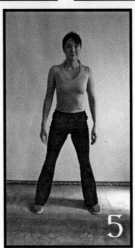

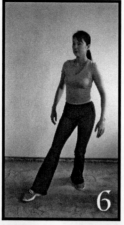
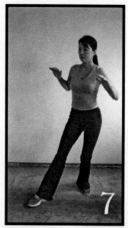
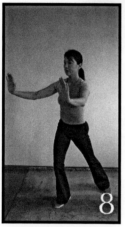
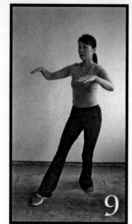
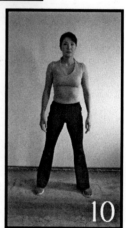

1. With knee bent, extend other leg forward diagonally.
2. Raise both wrists, keeping leg out in front.
3. Push palms all the way forward, while transferring body weight onto front foot.
4. Retract wrists back towards body, palms facing downwards.
5. Bring legs back to original position.
6. Repeat with opposite leg.
7. Raise both wrists, keeping leg out in front.
8. Extend palms all the way forward, while transferring body weight onto front foot.
9. Retract wrists back towards body, palms facing downwards.
10. Stand straight.

Number 11. A swan spreading its wings (Connecting the Pericardium Meridian)

Pericardium Meridian.: This route regulates the heart.

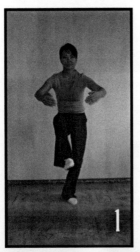
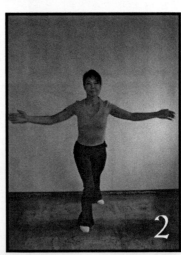
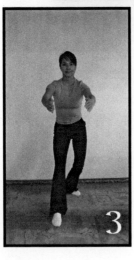
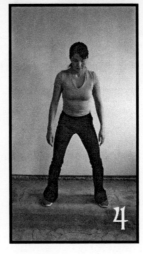
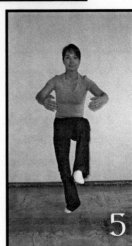

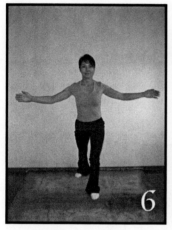 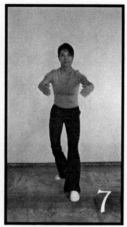 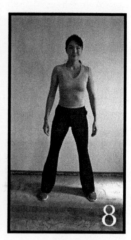

1. While raising one leg and bending the other, raise both arms above head, as if holding a ball.

2. Extend raised leg out in front to touch the floor, and transfer weight onto it, with arms extended out in front, palms facing forwards.

3. Slowly bring arms towards each other, transferring weight onto bent back leg.

4. Bring legs back towards standing position

5. Raise opposite leg, palms facing each other.

6. Repeat step 2, the other way around

7. Repeat step 3, the other way around.

8. Adopt standing position

Number 12. Bird's flight
(Connecting the Gall Bladder Meridian)

Gall Bladder Meridian: In conjunction with the liver meridian, this route regulates the gall bladder.

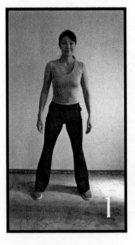 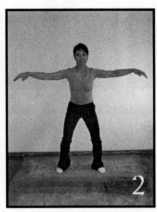 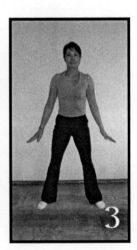

1. standing position.
2. Bending both knees, lower hips and raise both arms, palms facing downwards.
3. Straighten both legs, bring both arms down.

NUMBER 13. TURNING A WHEEL OF LIGHT (CONNECTING THE LIVER MERIDIAN)

This route regulates the liver, and the circulation.

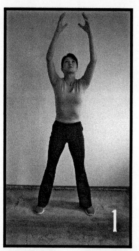
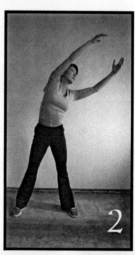
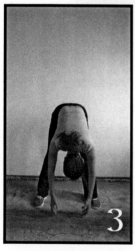
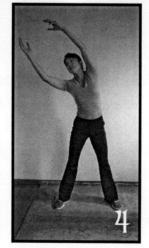
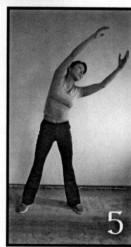

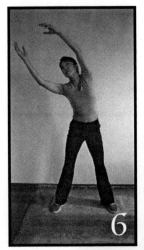 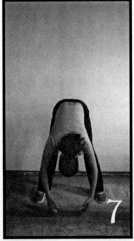 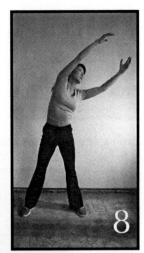

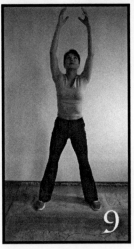 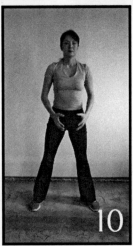

1. Raise both arms above head, as if holding a ball.

3. Rotate upper body all the way down without changing position of hips.

3. Continue slowly rotating until completely bent double.

4. Continue slowly rotating

5. Stop rotating when you have reached this diagonal position.

6. Now rotate in the other direction.

7. Repeat step 3

8. Continue rotating in this direction, palms facing each other.

9. Stop rotating, holding arms above head

10. Bring arms down slowly still as if holding a ball, to rest above abdomen.

NUMBER 14. RAISING AND LOWERING A BALL OF LIGHT (CONNECTING THE DU MERIDIAN AND THE REN MERIDIAN)

The Ren Meridian (or Conception Vessel): Mainly controlling the route at the front part of the body, in particular this regulates conception

The.Du Meridian: This oversees the body's spinal route, complementing the Ren Meridian , and regulating the brain.

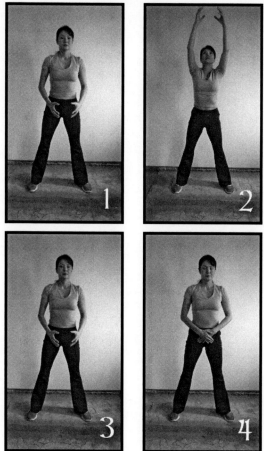

1. holding a ball, to rest above abdomen.
2. Raise both arms above head slowly, as if holding a ball.
3. Bring arms down slowly, still as if holding a ball, to rest above abdomen.
4. Men should place right hand on navel, women should place left, with the other hand placed on top.

MEDITATION

BECOME ONE WITH THE UNIVERSE.

Through learning the actual meaning of your life and your personal essence, you are presented with a fantastic chance to conquer your current circumstances. The deep mental training offered by the various practices of meditation enable us to vanquish self-hatred and see through life obstacles. Self-love results. Meditation allows the taking of a mental inventory. Through meditation we can go beyond the restricted framework that we call our *self*, and connect with the greater consciousness of the universe. Reaching a universal consciousness that transcends mere self-consciousness, we are brought into contact with an immense force through which miraculous healing can occur.

MEDITATION FOR HEALING

Practice meditation at times when you are in states of deep-level consciousness, usually this either before sleeping at night or upon waking in the morning. It is important to remove anything tight like ties, belts or bras. If possible try and get hold of some nice slow meditation music to have on in the background. If you are cold when you lie down on the bed, then get under the covers.

All sorts of reactions are likely to come out during meditation. To name a few, the constant prattle and dialogue in your head won't cease, you can't stop fretting, you may sneeze, feel aches and pains, slight choking, and saliva may come out. You might feel panicky, or have a sense of pent up frustration, and lethargy or a vacant mind are not uncommon. In fact, some people encounter extreme hot and cold spells, irrational fear, and sometimes dizziness. These sorts of disturbances are bound to arise during a meditation session at some point or other. If you find things to be unbearable then stop practicing meditation that day. It means that you must allow more time to advance, so just allow that. However, with practice you will eventually find yourself increasingly able to enter a meditative state. Through acquired strength gained over time and gentle but consistent perseverance you will discover that you are gradually healing yourself.

IMAGE OF MEDITATION CARRIED OUT FACING UPWARDS.

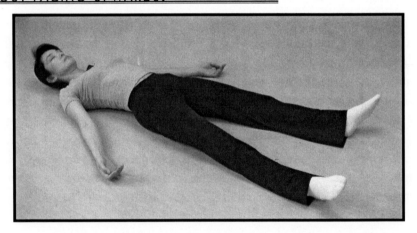

- First of all, lie down facing the ceiling, and stretch both legs, slightly parting them.

  Have your arms facing diagonally downward, with the palms of your hands facing upwards. Let go of any tension or power being held in your body and practice the breathing techniques over and over again. Close your eyes and relax while you are doing this.

- Try to feel both the senses and also a general repose within your body. If you feel like your body position might be imbalanced on any particular spot, adjust the way you are positioned so that your weight is evenly distributed as best possible.

- Feel the area around your forehead begin to warm up just slightly.

- This warmth moves from the top of the head to the face, and then around to the back of the head. A nice, comfortable feeling of ease ensues, and with it a sense of being very relaxed mentally.

- This warm, dozy feeling goes down to the neck, seeps into both arms, to the tips of the each finger, and then descends down to the chest. This mellow heavy feeling continues on further down the body and envelops the stomach, legs and feet going right to the tip of each toe.

- By now you will start to be feeling more and more deeply relaxed.
  At this point commence deep breathing. When you exhale, be sure to breathe out any negative thoughts or feelings from inside.

- Sense the parts of your body where you feel you are unwell or distressed. While breathing in and out feel the pain and tension within your body.

- Throughout the deep breathing, endeavor to hold in your mind the image of a white ball of light descending from above your head. . White and blue light is emanating from this ball, and shines as it engulfs your whole body. This is when the healing begins. The initial feeling is somewhat akin to having a large hand wrapped around your head.

- As the breathing gets slower and deeper, with it your body will relax increasingly.

- Consciously observe yourself, with the image of all of your pain and tension slipping away.

- As you continue the deep breathing, watch the blue and white light change to a gold colour, and then watch it flow into the areas of your body that require healing.

- You have conjured up this ball of light, and now entrust your body to it.

- The parts of your body that are suffering and the symptoms of illnesses are washed off and flow away from your body. They are then decomposed into gas, and disappear out of sight.
  While doing the deep breathing, do keep your ears tuned to the music that you have on.

- While you carry out the deep breathing, observe the healing process that you have just initiated. When you have completed in your mind the image of your problems being solved, and your ailments healed, it is time to begin slowly winding down the meditation session.

- Positively feel yourself lying down and relaxed in a safe place. It is an incredibly rich feeling. Keeping the breathing going steadily, slowly let yourself fall into a deep sleep. The healing continues even while you are asleep.

Bringing out and remedying problems and fears that have occurred in the past is something that takes time. Commit to yourself and persevere.

EPILOGUE

I was diagnosed with uterine cancer in 1991. Until then, I had always felt that I was above average in terms of health and strength and I felt that I had no connection whatsoever with serious illness. When the doctor diagnosed me with cancer, I felt the inside of my mind go completely blank, as many people say they do on hearing such news. There was no choice but to extract through surgery the organs that were afflicted by the cancer. How could it be, I asked myself as I plunged into the depths of depression, that I could have this illness when I was still single and hadn't even had children yet? I pitied my own existence.

The days leading up to the operation were grim and gloomy, and it seemed to rain perpetually. I was in and out of hospital, but was so despondent that I couldn't even bring myself to eat. It was at this point that a friend introduced me to a paranormal phenomenon healer who claimed to be able to beam a sort of energy onto the cancerous part of the body by placing hands over the area in question. By this stage I was open to anything, and so open I did make an appointment to see this healer for help. If I had been more blessed with time I would have liked to have received more of this treatment, but I got news that a bed was available in the hospital, and with that I promptly checked in.

After the operation, tests revealed that the cancer tumor first identified was getting a lot smaller than it had been before surgery. I questioned my doctor at the university hospital whether there had really been any need in the first place to be operated on.

He pointed out that I was speaking with the benefit of hindsight, and there have been many cases where patients with the same level of cancer as me had suffered a relapse and eventually died because of it.

I was dismayed that if I only had had more courage and time, I could have been healed merely through the paranormal phenomenon healing. All this was after the operation had taken place so there was really no more to be gained by obsessing about what might have been.

That said, I am eternally grateful to that healer, as thanks to him I was able to completely rid myself of all my stress and anxiety before the operation, and check into hospital in a remarkably positive frame of mind.

What the illness taught me was that everything in life happens for a reason, on a timely schedule, and is not merely coincidental. Our so-called "bad" experiences are not to be seen as wasted life experiences. Things occur as a result of cause and effect, and even when we are in the absolute depths of misery, experiences like illness are a precious learning experience that no doubt serves to teach and nurture both oneself and others.

On being discharged from hospital, I was resolved never to succumb to cancer again, and coupled with this decided to take up Qi Gong as a way of helping other people in the midst of suffering themselves. Not long afterwards, I happened to be at an event organized by the Japan Qi Gong Association where I was introduced to a young Chinese Qi Gong Teacher. This encounter was a starting point, as the following year together with some other Chinese doctors I ended up going on to open up a Qi Gong treatment centre. I was at first overwhelmed by the initial challenge of running a business, but also had the strong desire to help others, so endured. The fact that I had made the transition from being a hospital-bound patient a few months earlier to being part of the treatment sphere itself was beyond my imagination. Yet going with the natural flow of things, I even ended up going to a Chinese Massage School, studied Oriental Medicine in China and eventually progressed to a point where I myself was advising patients to undergo surgery and operations.

Since then, for some ten years or more I have been on the frontline of these things, and through seeing a large number of clients, realized the following. It seems that even if an illness is kept at bay by surgery, a patient will never be completely free of illness as long as responsibility for health is completely placed in the hands of the surgeon. I doubt that an illness would ever disappear while one is fundamentally dependant on a doctor.

Of course, as someone who has been there myself, in the case of a serious and potentially fatal illness it is prudent to entrust oneself to an expert in the field of that particular illness. One needs the help of a specialist when the energy of the body recedes. However, no matter how famous the doctor, therapist or healer is, they are merely a temporary medium for helping us.

The natural healing ability that we all posses is a healing energy that has been passed on to us from the gods and heavens above, and if we can strive to properly harness this inner power, we should definitely be able to use it to enact positive change in any circumstances. If you want to find the most deft and skillful doctor for you, then take a look in the mirror.

With medical expenses going up, and the ageing population advancing, we are at a time of great anxiety with regard to health. Becoming ill means incurring a huge mental and physical burden. If we are to deem health an essential asset for our precious lives, first of all it is incumbent upon us to re-program our thoughts and the deeds that govern our lifestyle. It is indispensable that we carry out mind-body maintenance on a daily basis in order to prolong and keep our good health. Qi Gong is a tower of strength for helping us to achieve this.

The sight of somebody striving to grow mentally, physically and spiritually through daily care for his or her precious life and body is a sight of sparkling beauty. In ancient times, it was believed that on dying we all ascend into the universe, returning to it as shining stars. In order to do so, one needed to gather up the amount of light necessary to shine in the sky above, or one would not be able to make the ascent. With Qi Gong as your tool, purify your heart and mind and send the light up high.

Make your own self into something burning, shining and bright!

Keiko Murakumo

Lightning Source UK Ltd.
Milton Keynes UK
28 November 2009

146874UK00001B/342/P